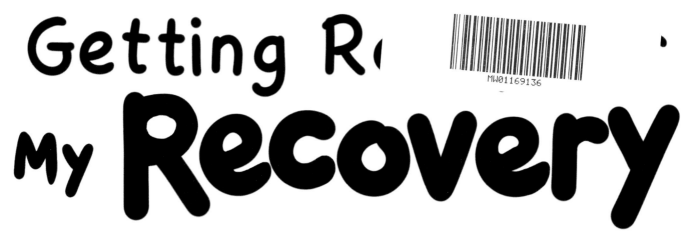

Getting Ready My Recovery

Surgery Recovery Book for Kids – From Hospital to Home

This book belongs to:

_____

Written by Dr. Fei Zheng-Ward   Illustrated by Moch. Fajar Shobaru

Copyright © 2025 Fei Zheng-Ward

Identifiers: ISBN 979-8-89318-080-0 (eBook)
ISBN 979-8-89318-081-7 (paperback)
ISBN 979-8-89318-082-4 (hardcover)

My surgery will be on my _____.
(write the body part above)

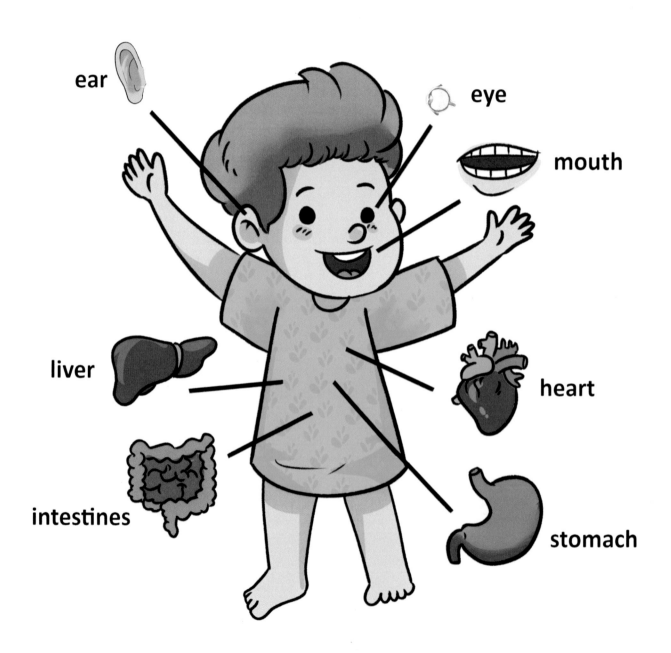

Or circle the part of the body where you will need surgery.

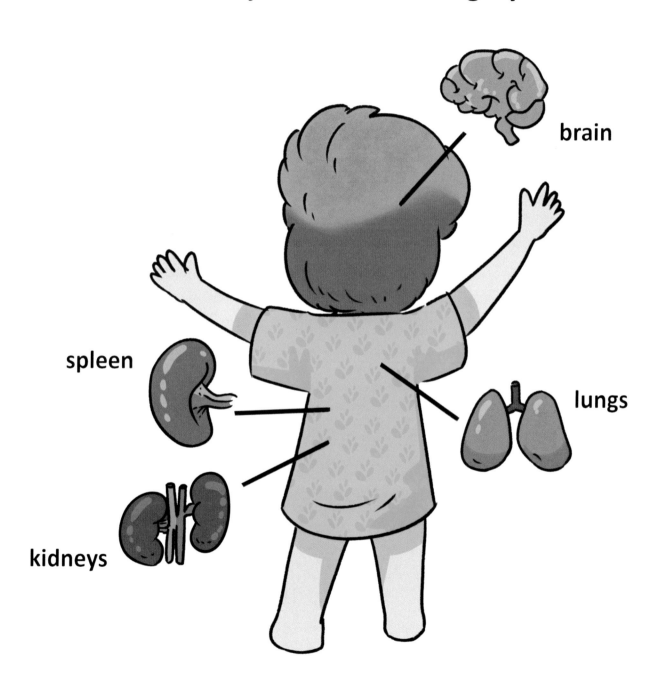

After your surgery, you will wake up in the hospital recovery room. You may feel uncomfortable, sore, or achy.

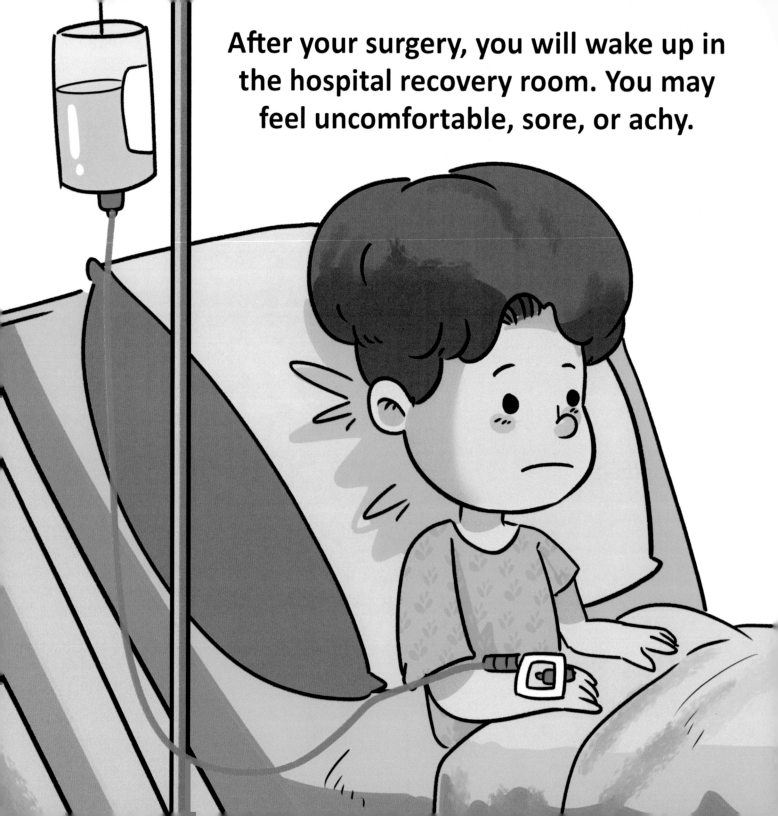

But don't worry, your nurse will give you medicine through the tiny plastic straw in your arm or leg to help you feel better.

The tiny straw, called an intravenous or IV catheter, was placed while you were asleep during your surgery.
It helps give your body a drink, lets your nurse give you special medicine to help you feel better, and allows your doctor to check your blood to make sure you're healing well.

What color IV catheter will you get?
Circle your color below.

yellow   **blue**   pink   green   gray   orange

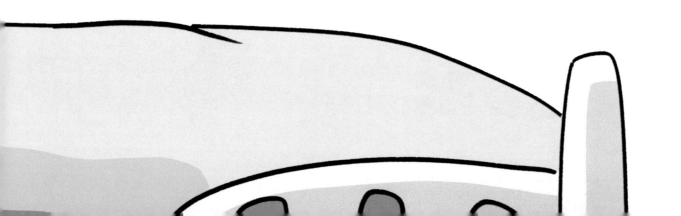

You may feel sick to your stomach,

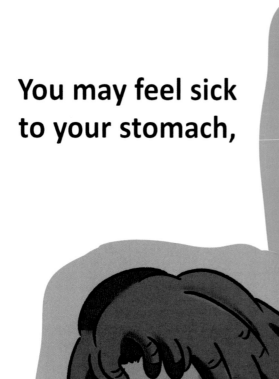

have a sore throat,

or feel a little dizzy or sleepy.

All of these feelings are normal after surgery and will get better soon.

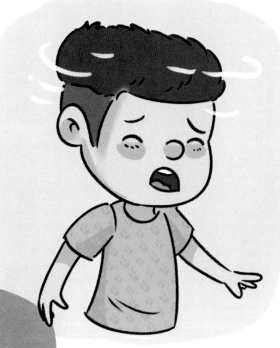

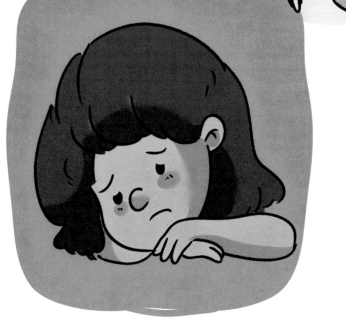

What are some things that can help you feel better after your surgery?

If something hurts, point to the thumb(s) or number below that shows how you feel.

This helps your nurse give you the right amount of medicine to help you feel better.

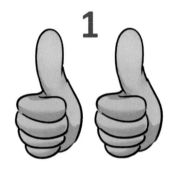

1

No pain

(I'm feeling good and
do NOT need pain
medicine)

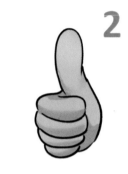

2

Tiny pain

(I'm feeling OK and do not
have to have pain medicine)

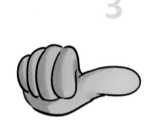

3

Some more pain

(I do need some pain medicine)

4

Even more pain

(I need MORE pain medicine)

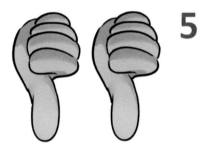

5

Worst pain

(I need MUCH MORE pain medicine NOW!)

You can rest with your favorite blanket or toy.

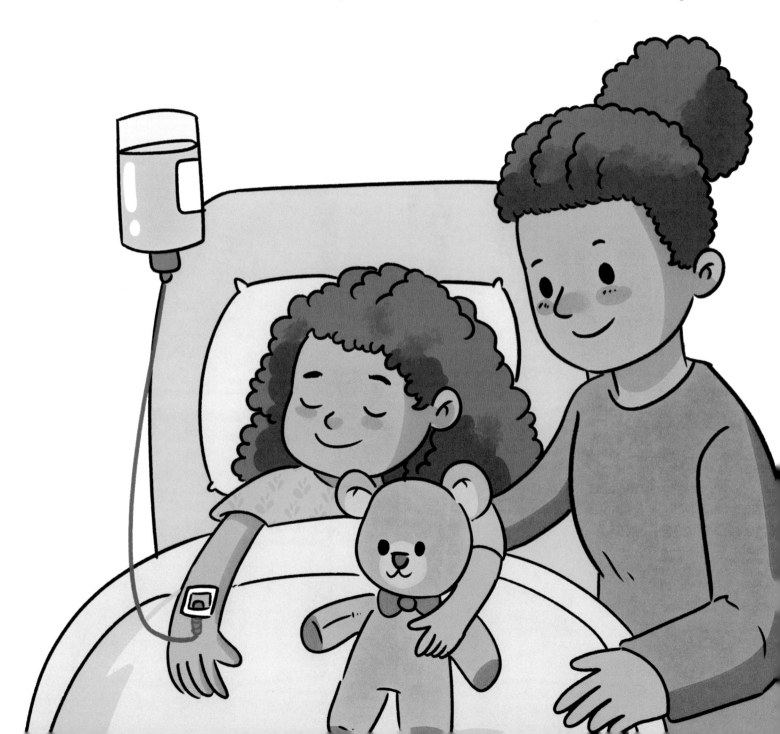

Depending on your surgery, you may see some tubes coming out of your body.
These tubes help your doctor and nurse take care of you and help you get better faster.

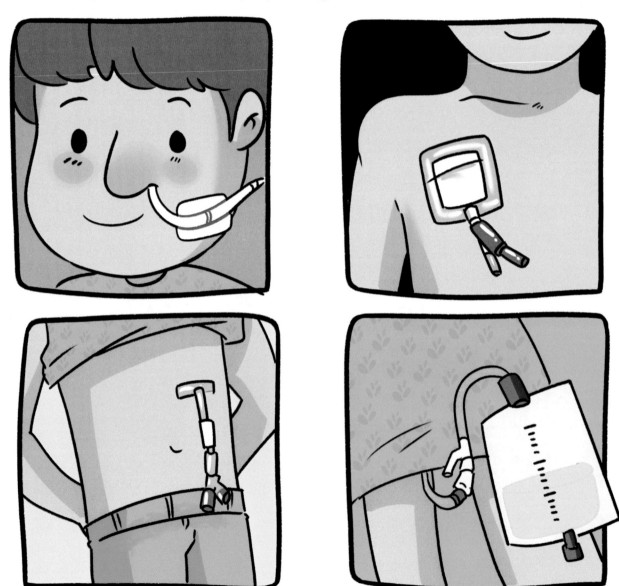

The tubes will be removed when you get stronger.
If your surgery was for a broken arm or leg,
you might have a cast to help it heal.

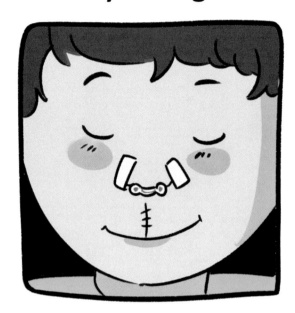

*You are
so brave!*

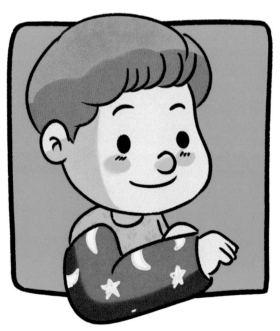

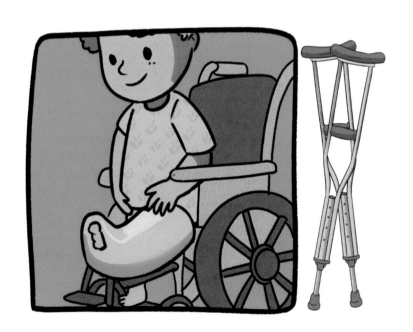

What helps you feel better?
Circle your answer(s) below.

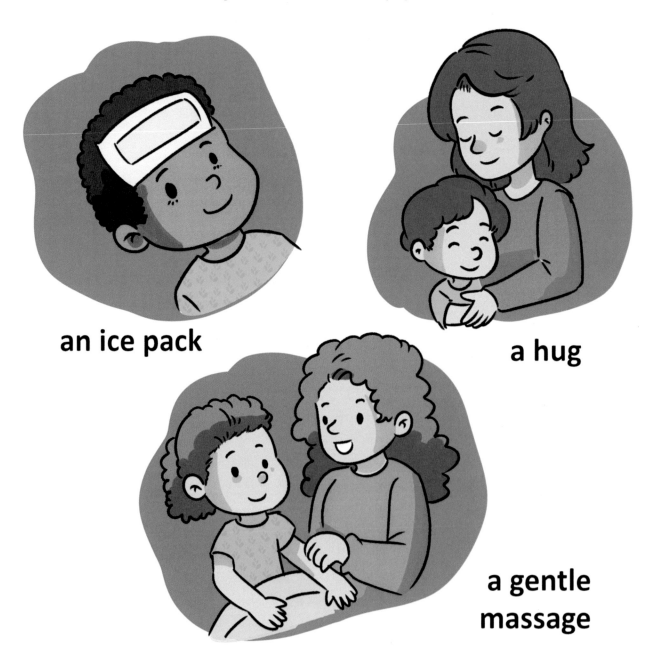

an ice pack

a hug

a gentle massage

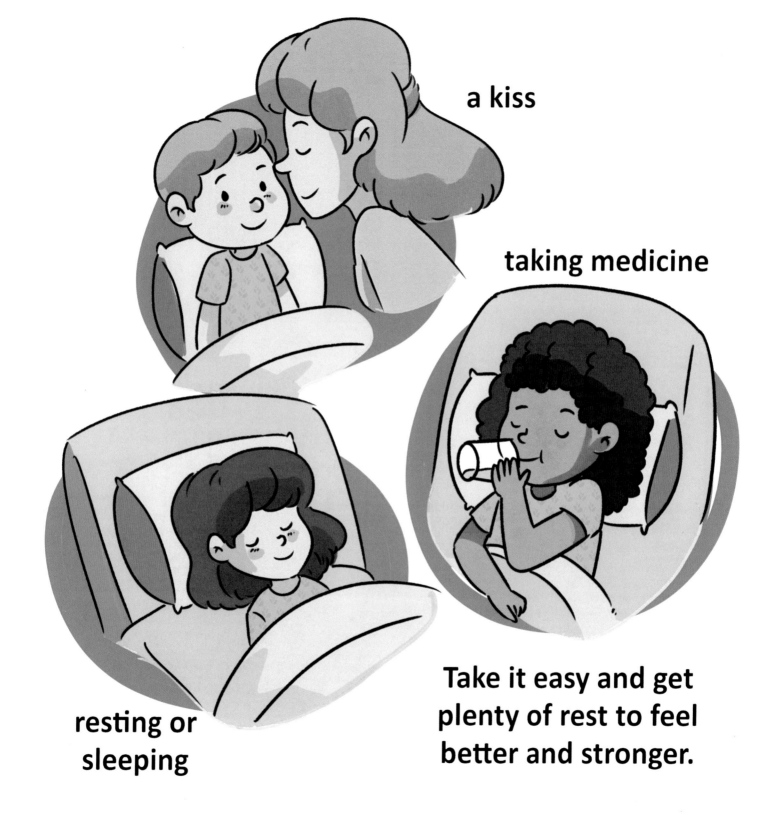

a kiss

taking medicine

resting or sleeping

Take it easy and get plenty of rest to feel better and stronger.

While you're in the recovery room, your doctor and nurse will check on you to make sure you're feeling okay.

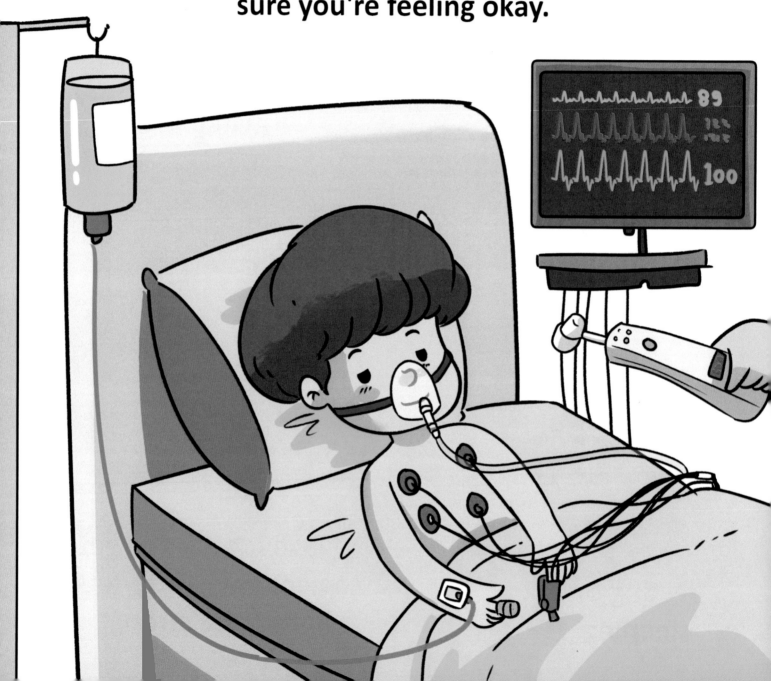

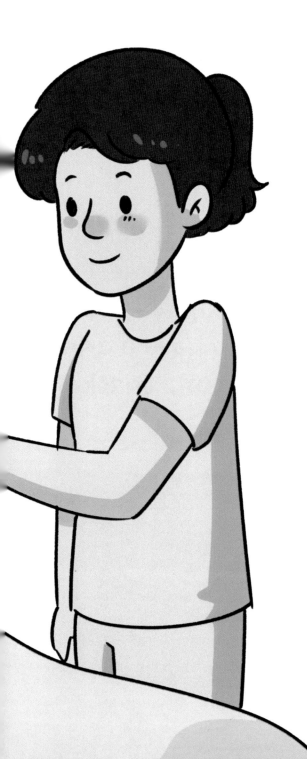

They will check your temperature, blood pressure, breathing, heart rate, and oxygen level in your body.

Every now and then, your doctor or nurse will check the part of your body that had surgery to make sure it's healing well and that your bandage is staying clean.

Sometimes, your nurse or doctor will help change your bandage to a new one.

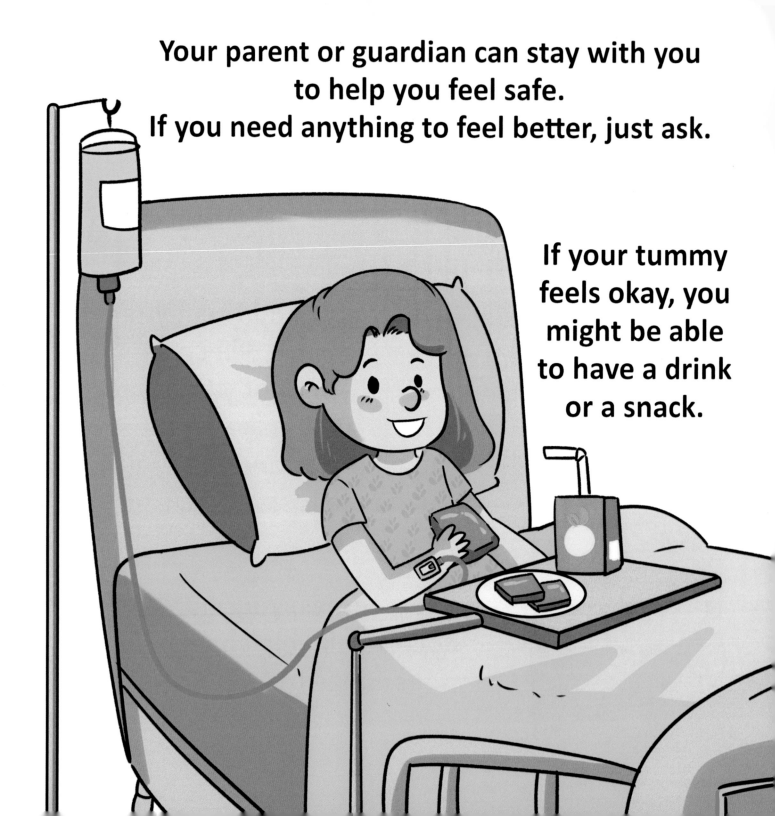

Your parent or guardian can stay with you
to help you feel safe.
If you need anything to feel better, just ask.

If your tummy
feels okay, you
might be able
to have a drink
or a snack.

Start with a sip of water or apple juice, or maybe a popsicle.

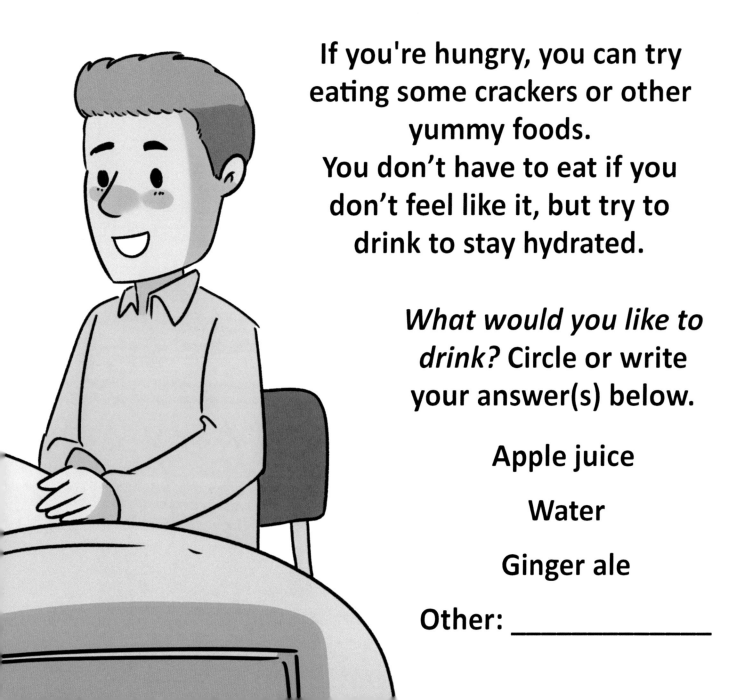

If you're hungry, you can try eating some crackers or other yummy foods.
You don't have to eat if you don't feel like it, but try to drink to stay hydrated.

What would you like to drink? Circle or write your answer(s) below.

Apple juice

Water

Ginger ale

Other: _____

Sometimes, you may need to spend the night at the hospital before going home.

You will get your own room, and your grown-up can stay with you to help you feel safe and comfortable.

Let's take a look at the special room they've prepared just for you.

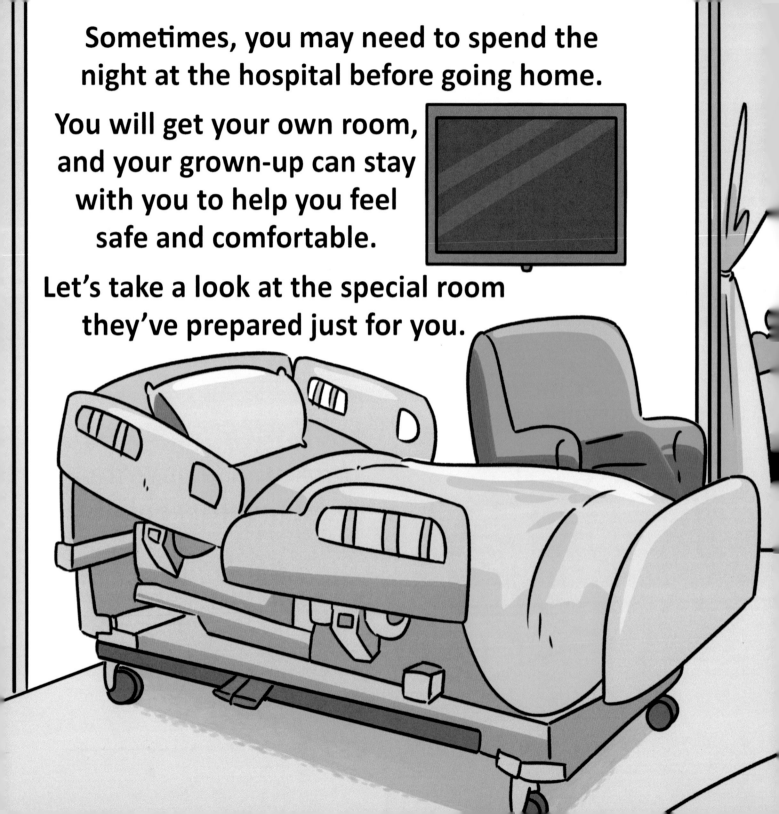

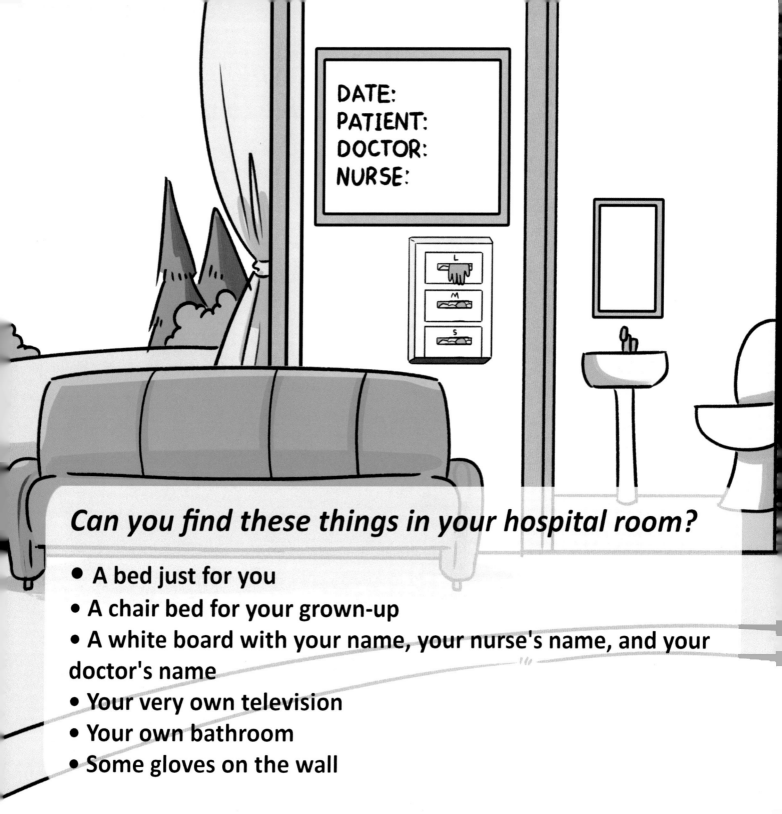

DATE:
PATIENT:
DOCTOR:
NURSE:

Can you find these things in your hospital room?

- A bed just for you
- A chair bed for your grown-up
- A white board with your name, your nurse's name, and your doctor's name
- Your very own television
- Your own bathroom
- Some gloves on the wall

While you recover in your room, what would you like to do?

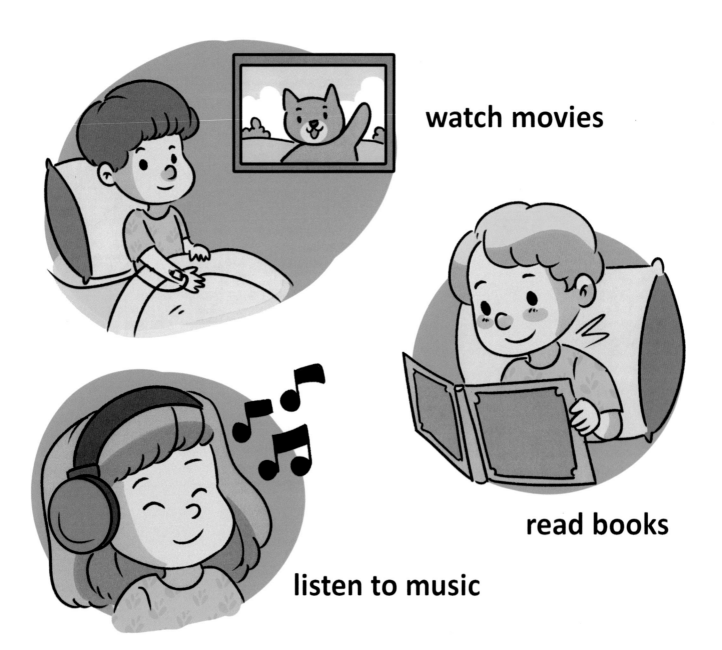

watch movies

read books

listen to music

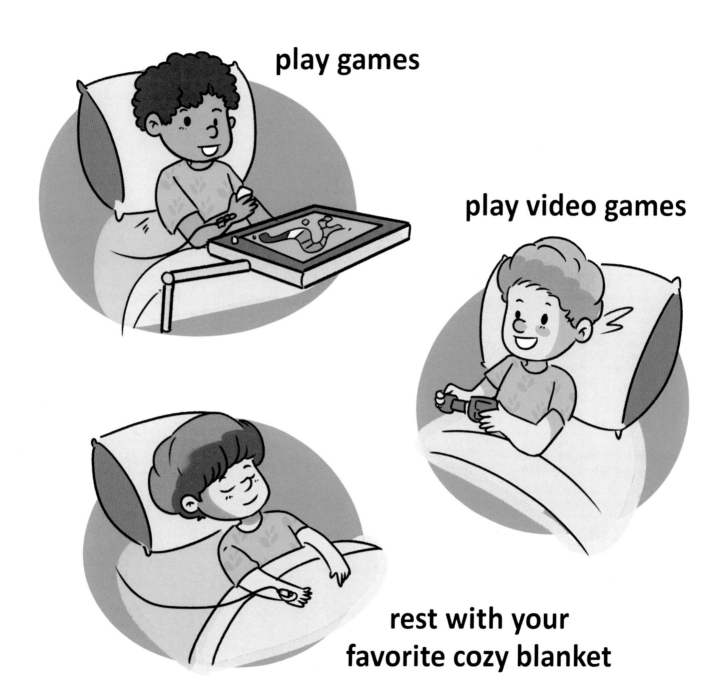

play games

play video games

rest with your
favorite cozy blanket

When you feel well enough, you can sit up in bed or in a chair.

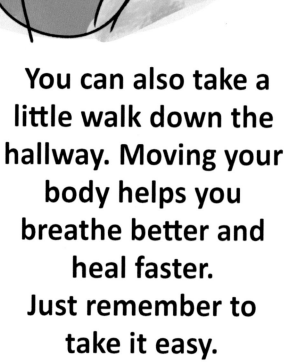

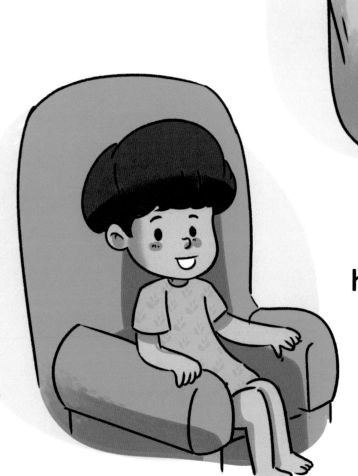

You can also take a little walk down the hallway. Moving your body helps you breathe better and heal faster.
Just remember to take it easy.

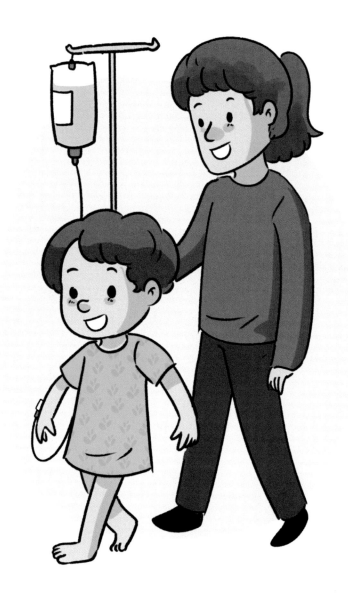

If you're getting out of bed, be sure to ask
your grown-up or nurse for help.

When you feel better and stronger, you'll be able to continue your recovery at home.

If you want to move around at home, please ask your parent or guardian to help you.

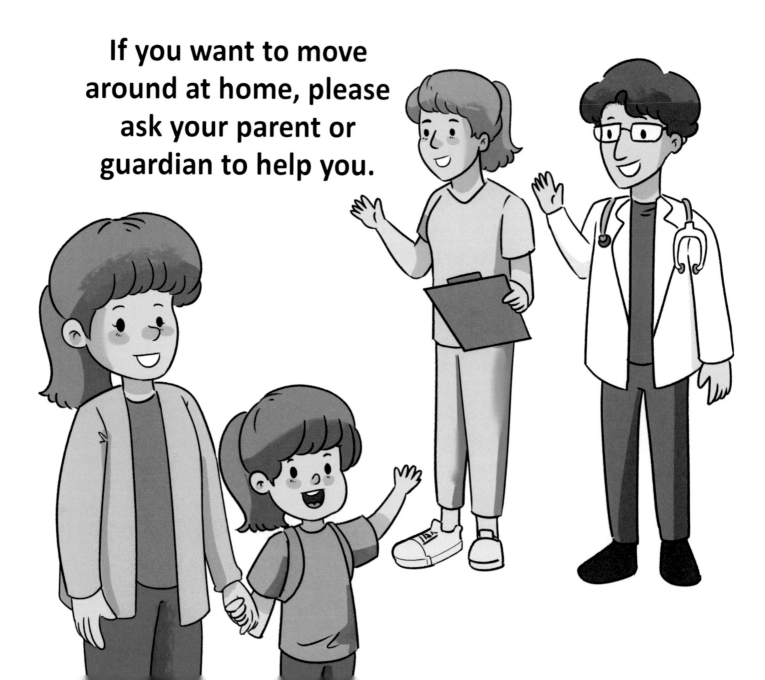

What are some fun things you can do at home to help you feel better? Circle the ones you like.

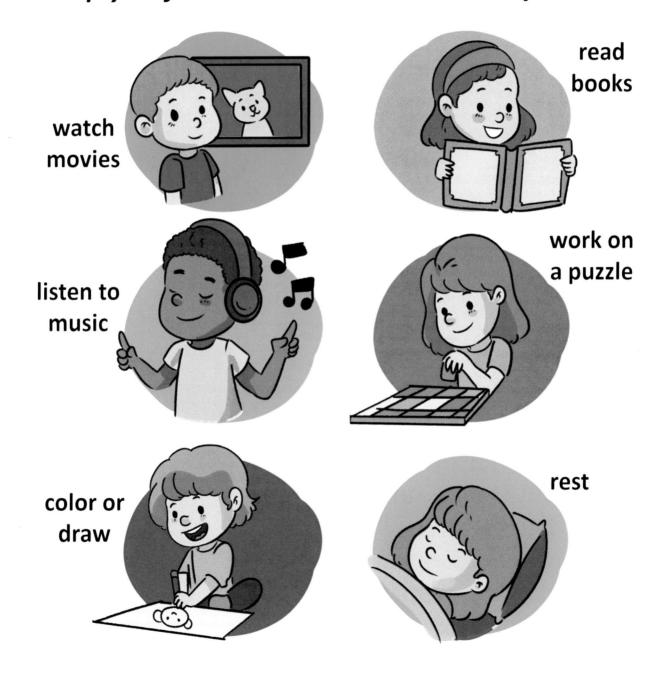

watch movies

read books

listen to music

work on a puzzle

color or draw

rest

Soon, you'll see your doctor again to make sure you're healing and feeling better.

If you have any questions, your doctor is happy to help.

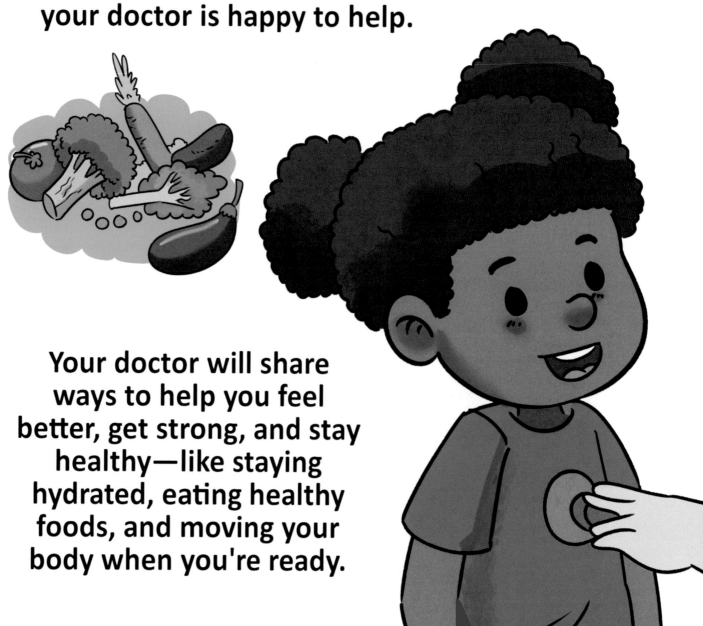

Your doctor will share ways to help you feel better, get strong, and stay healthy—like staying hydrated, eating healthy foods, and moving your body when you're ready.

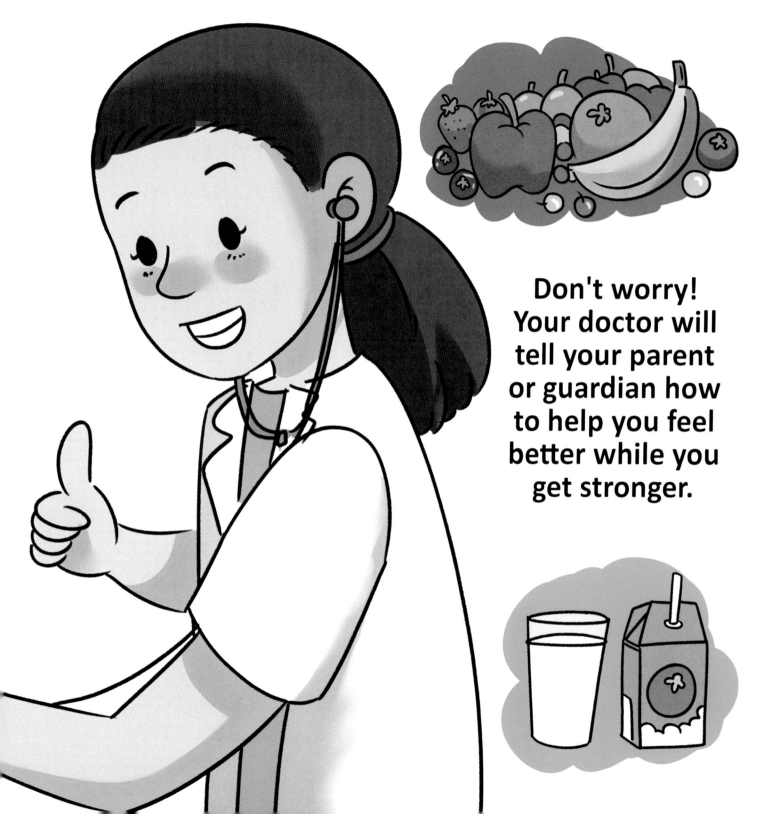

Don't worry! Your doctor will tell your parent or guardian how to help you feel better while you get stronger.

Before you know it, you'll be all better and ready to do the things you love again!

After recovery, how will you celebrate?
Draw or write your party plan below.

Speedy recovery!!

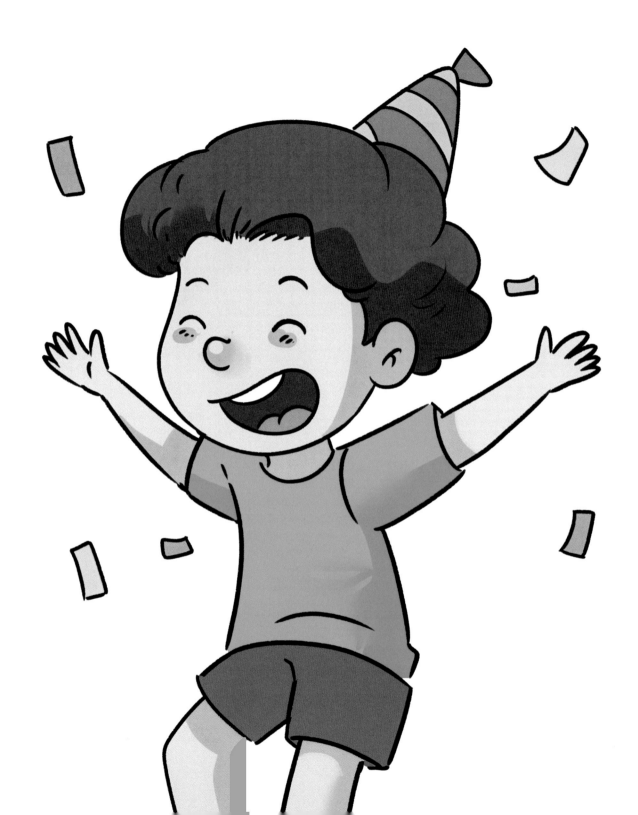

Notes for Parent/Guardian

- Placement of the intravenous (IV) catheter in this young age group is typically done _after_ your child is asleep in the operating room.

- After the surgery, it is common for children to feel confused, disoriented, or irritable, and they may cry, sob, kick, scream, or thrash around.
It normally takes about one hour for the anesthesia to wear off.

- Post-surgery instructions/restrictions:
Your child's doctor should give you specific instructions on (1) what your child can and cannot do during the recovery period, (2) the duration of the post-surgical restrictions, and (3) any post-surgical follow-ups. Additionally, (4) they should instruct what to watch out for and when it is necessary for you to bring your child back to the hospital in case of an emergency.
If they forget, please kindly remind them and obtain these instructions/restrictions before leaving the hospital.

Disclaimer

Please note that the illustrations are not drawn to scale.

This book is written for informational, educational, and personal growth purposes and should not be used as a substitute for medical advice.

Please consult your child's doctor if they need medical attention and to ensure the information in this book pertains to your child's medical condition and needs. I cannot guarantee what your child experiences is exactly what is being discussed in this book.

The author and the publisher are not responsible, either directly or indirectly, for any damages, monetary losses, or reparations due to information in this book. By reading this book, the readers agree not to hold the author and the publisher responsible for any losses as a result of any errors, inaccuracies, or omissions in this book.

Please keep in mind that your child's experience depends on the location, the facility, their medical condition, and the healthcare team. Please use this book in conjunction with your child's doctor's advice. Thank you.

Did this picture book help your child in some way?
If so, I would love to hear about it!

www.amazon.com/gp/product-review/B0F8RCZDFV

For other book titles, please visit:

www.fzwbooks.com

Connect with the author

email: books@fzwbooks.com
facebook/instagram: @FZWbooks

About the Author

Dr. Fei Zheng-Ward is a clinical anesthesiologist who understands the apprehension patients (both adults and children) may have surrounding their upcoming surgery. Her goal in her medical books is to bring useful information to patients so they have a better understanding and appreciation of what happens leading up to, during, and after surgery. She wants readers to be more empowered to make informed decisions and to feel more at ease with their surgery.

As a practicing physician, she takes pride in being respected for her attention to detail, commitment to providing compassionate and personalized patient care, and strong presence in patient advocacy in the perioperative period for each of her patients. She understands the importance of physical and emotional well-being and advocates for patient autonomy.

Her other children's books aim to bring laughter into your family, encourage children to be more helpful at home, and inspire a love of reading.

She is an award-winning author for her book titled ***What to Expect and How to Prepare for Your Surgery***.

More about Dr. Fei Zheng-Ward:

• Board Certified Anesthesiologist

• Anesthesiology Residency Training at The Johns Hopkins Hospital in Baltimore, MD

• Master in Public Health (MPH) degree from Dartmouth Medical School in Hanover, NH

FEI ZHENG-WARD, MD, MPH

WHAT TO EXPECT
and
HOW TO PREPARE
for Your
SURGERY

A PATIENT'S GUIDE TO UNDERGOING ANESTHESIA AND MORE!

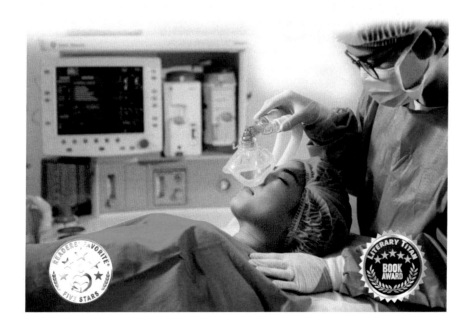

Books by the author

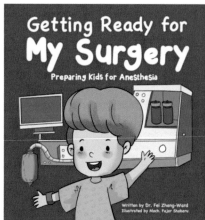

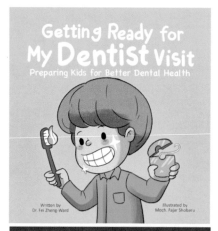

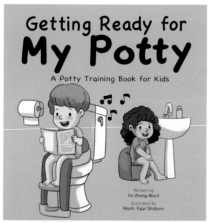

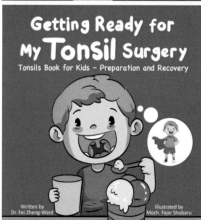

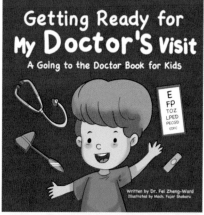

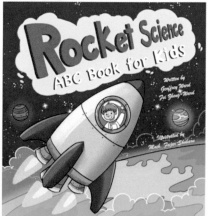

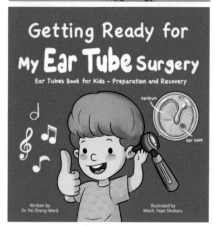

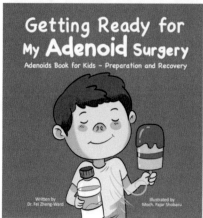

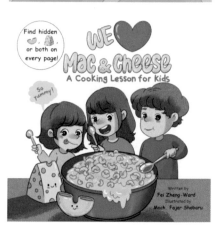

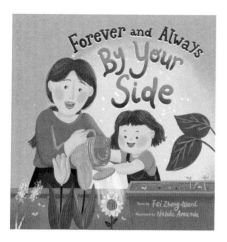

Forever and Always By Your Side
Story by Fei Zheng-Ward
Illustrated by Nabila Amanda

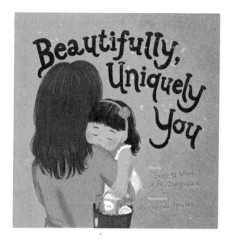

Beautifully, Uniquely You
Story by Geoffrey Ward & Fei Zheng-Ward
Illustrated by Nabila Amanda

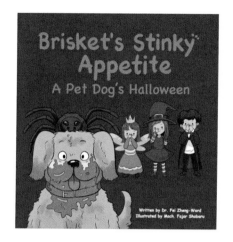

Brisket's Stinky Appetite
A Pet Dog's Halloween
Written by Dr. Fei Zheng-Ward
Illustrated by Mach. Fajar Shabaru

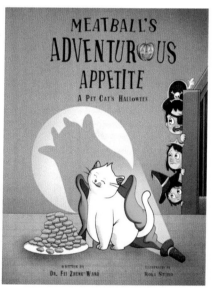

MEATBALL'S ADVENTUROUS APPETITE
A Pet Cat's Halloween
WRITTEN BY Dr. Fei Zheng-Ward
ILLUSTRATED BY Roka Studio

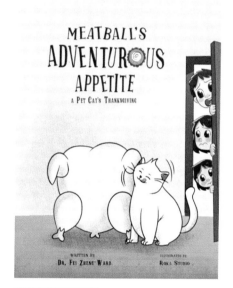

MEATBALL'S ADVENTUROUS APPETITE
A Pet Cat's Thanksgiving
WRITTEN BY Dr. Fei Zheng-Ward
ILLUSTRATED BY Roka Studio

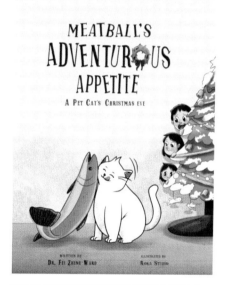

MEATBALL'S ADVENTUROUS APPETITE
A Pet Cat's Christmas Eve
WRITTEN BY Dr. Fei Zheng-Ward
ILLUSTRATED BY Roka Studio

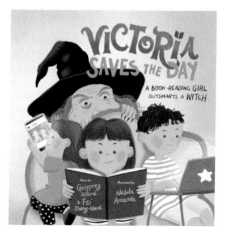

VICTORIA SAVES THE DAY
A BOOK-READING GIRL OUTSMARTS A WITCH
Story by Geoffrey Ward & Fei Zheng-Ward
Illustrated by Nabila Amanda

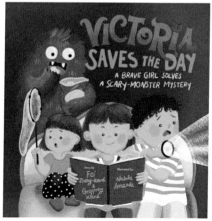

VICTORIA SAVES THE DAY
A BRAVE GIRL SOLVES A SCARY-MONSTER MYSTERY
Story by Fei Zheng-Ward & Geoffrey Ward
Illustrated by Nabila Amanda

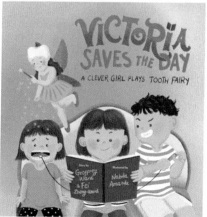

VICTORIA SAVES THE DAY
A CLEVER GIRL PLAYS TOOTH FAIRY
Story by Geoffrey Ward & Fei Zheng-Ward
Illustrated by Nabila Amanda

Made in the USA
Monee, IL
21 June 2025

19779631R00021